Eat, Drink
Be Well

The Alkaline Diet Choice
For Cancer Prevention

Published by Alkaline People Publishing
6352 Corte Del Abeto, Suite H
Carlsbad, CA 92011
800.662.0189
www.AlkalinePeoplePublishing.com

Printed in the United States
1st Printing July 2009

For questions or comments, please send correspondence to the above address.

These statements have not been evaluated by the food and drug administration. The preceding information and/or products are for educational purposes only and are not meant to diagnose, prescribe, or treat illness. Please consult your doctor before making any changes or before starting ANY exercise or nutritional supplement program or before using this information or any product during pregnancy or if you have a serious medical condition.

TABLE OF CONTENTS

Introduction

At the start of the 21st century, many scourges from the past are but distant memories. Polio, which killed over 3,000 Americans in 1955, is now almost unheard of the United States. Measles, mumps, rubella, typhoid, diphtheria, and other diseases that swept away millions are now prevented through improved sanitation, hygiene, and preventive care.

Yet one scourge remains: cancer.

Cancer is a scary word. The big "C" is a diagnosis no one wants to hear. Everyone knows someone who has been diagnosed with cancer or has died from cancer. Cancer, it seems, is everywhere. According to the American Cancer Society[1], 1.4 million new cases of cancer were diagnosed in the United States in 2008, the last year for which complete figures are available.

Cancer is a disease caused by the unchecked mutation and growth of cells within the body. It can strike nearly every organ and area of the body, from the brain and bones to the liver, kidney, pancreas, breast, bowel and uterus. Some cancers are silent killers, making their presence known only when it's too late, while others have a high survival rate.

Most cancers occur in people age 55 and older. As the body ages, it appears that in some people, the genetic code within specific cells becomes garbled or corrupted, much like computer code that degrades over time. As it degrades, it does not divide properly, leading to mutations that may in turn become cancerous.

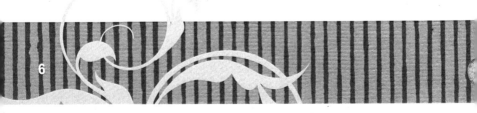

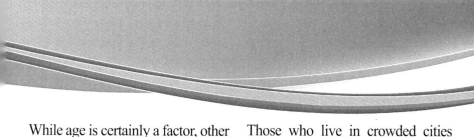

While age is certainly a factor, other factors come into play to assess cancer risk. The other important factors are heredity, environment, and lifestyle choices. Heredity means the genetic material we inherit from our parents and ancestors. The genetic deck is shuffled before conception, and fate hands us the cards we must play in life. Some cards make us tall or blue eyed, while others appear to make us prone to cancer, diabetes, and other disease. There's not much we can do about our heredity.

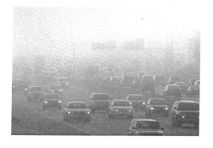

It's the last two factors, however, that seem to tip fate's hand into cancer if the cards we're dealt include cancer. Our environment from birth onwards can influence cancer risk.

Those who live in crowded cities breathing smog from car and bus exhaust may be more susceptible to cancer than those living at the top of a pristine mountain among the wildflowers. Environmental toxins, from polluted water to high levels of stress, may create the conditions necessary for cells to mutate into cancer.

Among all the factors affecting the likelihood of cancer, the one most in everyone's control is lifestyle. From the food you eat, to the water you drink, to the amount of exercise you get every day, and from choices like whether to smoke cigarettes or drink alcohol, lifestyle is entirely within the individual's control.

Here's what the American Cancer Society states about lifestyle factors:

Scientific evidence suggests that about one-third of the 565,650 cancer deaths expected to occur in 2008 will be related to over weight or obesity, physical inactivity, and nutrition and thus could also be prevented. Certain cancers are related to infectious agents, such as hepatitis B virus (HBV), human papillomavirus (HPV), human immunodeficiency virus (HIV), *Helicobacter pylori (H. pylori)*, and others, and could be prevented through behavioral changes. In addition, many of the more than 1 million skin cancers that are expected to be diagnosed in 2008 could have been prevented by protection from the sun's rays and avoiding indoor tanning.[2]

If we look at the 10 most common kinds of cancer among American women, for example, we see that the National Cancer Institute and the Center for Disease Control[3] lists the following as the top 10 most common cancers among women:

1. Breast Cancer (117.7)
2. Lung (and Bronchus) Cancer (54.2)
3. Colon and Rectal Cancer (42.7)
4. Corpus and Uterus, NOS (23.1)
5. Non-Hodgkin Lymphoma (16.1)
6. Skin Melanomas (14.0)
7. Thyroid Cancer (13.8)
8. Ovarian Cancer (12.5)
9. Kidney and Renal Pelvis Cancer (10.0)
10. Pancreatic Cancer (9.7)

Among these cancers, three can be prevented through lifestyle choices. Smoking cessation, increased fiber consumption through fruits and vegetables, and more exercise could prevent lung and colon cancer. Avoiding extremes in sunbathing, while still getting healthy doses of sunlight for vitamin D production, would lower the rate of skin melanomas.

Some would argue that nearly all could be prevented through significant lifestyle changes. That's where the acid-alkaline balance comes into the equation.

Chronic Acidosis as a Cause of Cancer

Think back to high school chemistry classes. Do you remember the pH scale? The pH scale refers to the concentration of hydrogen ions found within a substance. The scale[4] ranges from 0, the strongest acids known such as battery acid, to 14, an alkaline substance like drain cleaner that is also toxic. In fact, anything on the extreme ends of the pH scale is dangerous to life! The tipping point is a pH of 7, considered neutral. This is found in so-called pure water.

Within the human body, the pH of various bodily fluids changes. Stomach and gastric fluids are highly acidic, with a pH of 1 for the hydrochloric acid secreted by the stomach to blood pH, which is kept in a strict range at 7.35 – 7.45.

The foods that the average American eats range in the pH scale with most being acidic and some being alkaline. What happens to them when they enter the body? Take beef, for example. Beef is the most acidic meat on the entire food scale, with pork, veal, and chicken coming in right behind it. When you eat beef, it enters the stomach, where it is mixed with digestive juices. As the process of digestion unfolds, the meat throws the body into a slightly acidic state. The body rushes to buffer the excess acids. Again, think back to high school chemistry class. A buffer is a substance that neutralizes acid. Inside your body, such buffers are minerals like calcium. And where does that calcium come from? Well, if you are acidic, it comes from your own bones.

You may remember that calcium is one of the building blocks of bone health. The dairy lobbying industry exhorts everyone to drink their milk to build strong bones, yet Westerners have the highest rate of osteoporosis in the world. Asians, on the other hand, who drink little or no milk, have the lowest incidence of bone fractures associated with osteoporosis[5] What's going on?

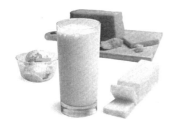

It's simple: almost all cows' milk and dairy products are on the acidic end of the scale. Any and all calcium entering the body is used to buffer all those acids. Along with it, the calcium already deposited in the bones is used to buffer the effects of the cows' milk and that means you end up with a negative calcium factor!

But the acid-alkaline problem affects more than just bone health, it also affects cancer rates.

Cancer Prevention through an Alkaline Diet

More and more research is pointing towards prevention as the key to beating cancer, rather than a magic vaccine, pill or panacea. The acid-alkaline balance is an important part of the equation. When the balance of the diet draws the body into an acidic state, it's predisposed to cancer. Shift the chemistry towards the alkaline end of the scale, and cancers cells struggle to survive.

In this book, we'll share with you the known links between various forms of cancer and what you eat.

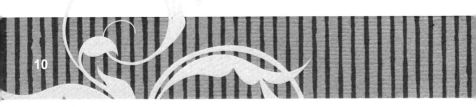

We'll share with you the latest research on which foods are known for cancer prevention, and which probably won't make a difference.

You'll learn the importance of eating not just cancer preventing foods, but foods that induce an alkaline state throughout the body. If you're still confused about what that means, don't worry—we'll review the basics again, why they're important, and how to easily and naturally create the alkalinity we believe is important to cancer prevention. Section 3 includes lots of information in short, digestible bites, along with charts and tables that are easy to use to help you get started on an alkaline, cancer–prevention diet.

Water is vital to health, yet not all water is created equal. Some water will actually support an alkaline lifestyle. You'll learn more about that in section 4.

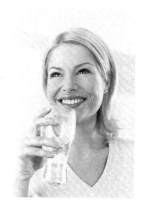

Other factors in your external and internal environment can lead to cancer. Some of these you know about already, like carcinogens in foods, asbestos in the air, pollution and exposure to chemicals. But did you know that long-term emotional stress can be toxic— or that you yourself can control your emotional state? It's true. You are what you think, and we'll help you with techniques to think positive, productive, life-affirming thoughts in section 5.

Lastly, because we know that not all your questions will be answered in one book, we've included a resource list. Read the origin of the studies cited in this report, or delve into the various websites that support an alkaline diet. Find alkaline water machines, alkaline foods, and other equipment to help you detoxify your home and lead a healthy, natural, and holistic life.

An old English proverb warns "Don't dig your grave with your knife and fork."[6] Instead of eating your way towards illness, choose the life-affirming foods of the alkaline diet.

Bon appetit!

Chapter One
Cancer and Diet: The Connection

As we noted in the introduction, many of today's most common cancers can be prevented—partially or entirely—through lifestyle changes.

Take lung cancer for example. The preponderance of evidence strongly suggests that smoking tobacco causes lung cancer. While exposure to pollution or toxins like asbestos may also cause cancer, the majority of lung cancer sufferers puffed their way into sickness.

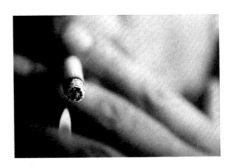

CANCERS RELATED TO LIFESTYLE AND DIET		
TYPE	CONTRIBUTING FACTOR *(in addition to genetics)*	PREVENTATIVE MEASURE
LUNG CANCER	Smoking or use of tobacco products	Do not smoke or chew tobacco
SKIN CANCER *(melanoma)*	Excessive sun exposure	Avoid prolonged sun exposure or sunburns and indoor tanning
BREAST CANCER	Foods rich in fats and oils	Eat a low fat diet, exercise
COLON CANCER	Foods high in meat, fats and oils	Switch to a Vegetarian, Vegan or Raw Food diet, eat low fat diet, exercise

Information above taken from "Major Killers," published by the Physician's Committee for Responsible Medicine with some additions by RawPeople.

Another so-called "lifestyle" cancer is skin cancer or melanoma. Many people broil themselves like steaks on the grill. While some sun exposure helps the body produce optimal amounts of vitamin D, overexposure, particularly since the world's protective layer of ozone is depleted, can lead to too much UVA and UVB rays that lead to skin cancer. Donning protective clothing and limiting sun exposure, or working outdoors morning or late afternoon, should suffice to protect most people from too much sun exposure.

The last two cancers may puzzle some people on the list of lifestyle cancers. Breast cancer and colon cancer seem to most people to strike at random. Scientists know that genetics plays a role in susceptibility to both cancers, with a strong familial connection and genetic markers for certain types of breast cancer.[7] But diet also influences the occurrence of both types of cancer.

High Fat Diets and the Link to Breast Cancer

A diet high in fat may dispose some women to breast cancer. That's the latest information from the National Cancer Institute, as reported on Web MD.[8]

According to the report, postmenopausal women who ate a high-fat diet were 15% more likely to develop breast cancer than women who consistently ate a low fat diet. The study followed over 180,000 women for four years.

Considering that the American Cancer Society predicts that in 2008 over 188,000 women will

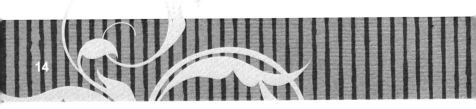

develop breast cancer, if we can prevent 15% of all breast cancers that means 28,200 women will be spared the agony of a breast cancer diagnosis!

Do dairy products cause breast cancer?

Dairy products have gotten a bad rap among those who study diet and cancer risk, particularly the link between dairy products and breast cancer. In addition to being high fat, dairy products such as milk frequently contain hormones and antibiotics fed to factory-farmed dairy cows. When ingested, such toxins may be stored in fatty tissues, such as the breast. While it's not definite, these factors— plus the highly acidic nature of dairy, as we'll discuss in section 3—may make dairy something to leave out of your diet if breast cancer is of particular concern.

Colon Cancer: Eat Your Vegetables

The colon is one of the most neglected organs of the body, yet it is one of the most important. This vital organ shuttles wastes from the body. Constipation isn't just an uncomfortable nuisance— it can actually be life threatening. The two most common causes of constipation are lack of fiber in the diet and dehydration. Both are very important to colon health.

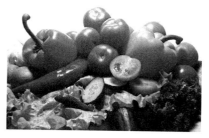

As food moves through the digestive system, it passed from the mouth to the stomach and then to the small intestine. Along the way, various nutrients are removed, along with water. What's left behind is material the body cannot use and fiber. Fiber comes in two forms: soluble and insoluble. Both fibers are found in nature and contribute to colon health and cancer prevention. Fibers bind with fatty acids and move food rapidly through the colon. Remember that the material moving into the colon contains elements the body cannot use for digestion. These can include any pesticide residue and chemical nasties that were in the food to begin with, and if the food moves rapidly, it has less contact with the colon walls. The less contact these toxins have, the less chance they have of influencing cell growth and division.

Foods to Prevent Colon Cancer:

Certain foods, particularly fruits and vegetables, contain compounds thought to ward off colon cancer. The American Cancer Society recommends eating the following foods to prevent colorectal cancer:

- Green leafy vegetables, such as spinach, kale, and Swiss chard
- Brussels sprouts
- Broccoli
- Fruits high in fiber, such as berries, cantaloupes, papayas and dried apricots
- Whole grains, which are rich in both fiber and nutrients

While colorectal cancer is a combination of genetic predisposition and diet, the American Cancer Society estimates that approximately 75% of all diagnosed cases of colorectal cancer are diet related. Obesity, which is often the result of a poor diet or a diet high in fats, appears to be a leading contributing factor in many cancers but especially colorectal cancer.

What We Know About Food: Cancer and Diet

Based on these scary statistics, it seems as if many of the foods you love cause cancer, or contribute to weight gain that appears linked with cancer.

Weight Gain and the Acidic Diet

Before we move on and talk more about diet, let's talk a little about how an acidic diet encourages weight gain. Keep in mind that too much acid is bad for the body, and the body will try to protect itself from too much acid. It does this by either getting rid of the acid, or storing it, much the way it can store toxins that it can't dispose of properly. The body will store these acids in the tissues and surround them with water and fat. Thus, a highly acidic diet encourages the body to put on fat – while switching to a more alkaline diet encourages weight loss. Many people who switch to an alkaline diet are surprised by the rapid weight loss. If your weight stubbornly refuses to budge, try an alkaline diet. You may be surprised. Your body will be grateful that it can shed all the excess fat, water, and acidic waste.[10]

Free Radicals:

You may have heard that antioxidants are important in the fight against cancer because they protect against free radicals. Free radicals are atoms or molecules or ions with an unpaired outer shell electron. They bounce around inside the cells and seek an atom that they can steal the electron from. This turns the atom it steals from into a free radical. The result is damage to a cell's DNA, which affects either how the cell replicates, or recreates itself, or how quickly the cell recreates itself. Both results are precancerous conditions or cancer. Antioxidants are potent chemicals that mop up free radicals before they have the chance to damage cells. They're abundant in richly colored fruits and vegetables like grapes, tomatoes, and more. It's best to get them from foods and not from pills or supplements. Vitamins C and E can donate an electron, which makes them strong antioxdants. Another great source of antioxidants is from ionized alkaline mineral water that is created from water ionizer machines.

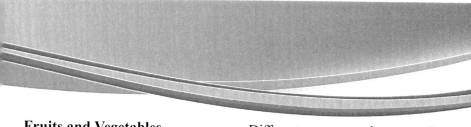

Fruits and Vegetables

Fruits and vegetables are the heavy lifters in the body's daily defense against cancer. They contain important chemicals called phytochemicals that help protect the body against free radical damage that leads to cancer.

What are phytochemicals?[11] Phyto-chemicals are compounds found within plants. They contain antioxidants, some hormones, and chemicals that stimulate enzymes. They can interfere with DNA replication, which is important in the fight against cancer. Some phytochemicals, such as the ones found in garlic, have natural antibacterial properties. Others prevent the bad stuff like bacteria from sticking to cell walls. Cranberries are one such example. Drinking unsweetened cranberry juice can treat or prevent the bacteria that cause bladder infections from adhering to the bladder cell walls.

Different compounds naturally occur in different plants. Broccoli, cabbage, Brussels sprouts and other strong-tasting vegetables are rich in compounds called indoles. These stimulate estrogen-blocking enzymes, which are important in the fight against estrogen-fueled cancers, such as breast and uterine cancer. Other plants contain powerful antioxidants that battle cancer differently. Tomatoes contain lypocene[12], a compound that facilitates the transformation of beta carotene into vitamin A in the body, among other things, and a compound now studied in the quest to find a preventative for prostate cancer.

As you can see, phytochemicals pack one powerful punch in the fight against cancer. While supplement manufacturers continue to try to distill these cancer and disease fighters into a pill, the best source of phytochemicals remains fresh fruits and vegetables.

Eat a Rainbow a Day

Fill your plate with a rainbow of fruits and vegetables each day!

Apples, Strawberries

Oranges, Acorn Squash

Squash

Green Leafy Vegetables

Blueberries

Grapes, Plums, Beets

Whole Grains

Life fruits and vegetables, whole grains—grains that contain the germ, or outer covering of the seed part, as well as the inner portion—are rich in phytochemicals. They're also chock full of fiber, an important addition to the diet that helps ward off colorectal cancer. When considering grains, look for "brown" grains as opposed to "white" or refined grains. White rice and white flour, for example, are lifeless and stripped of all the healthful benefits of their whole grain counterparts. And don't limit yourself to rice and wheat; there's delicious quinoa, spelt, and myriad other whole grains in the aisles of your supermarket or local health food store. While quinoa may not be technically a grain, it's cooked like one, so most people call it a grain. It's also a complete source of protein and contains all eight essential amino acids.

Wheat grass juice

Another potent alkaline diet aid and anti-cancer food is wheatgrass juice.

What is Wheatgrass Juice?

Wheatgrass is exactly what it sounds like – the young sprouts of hard red winter wheat. Grass is harvested and juiced. The resulting liquid is highly alkalizing, as well as detoxifying.

Ann Wigmore and Wheatgrass

We can't mention wheatgrass without mentioning Ann Wigmore. A passionate natural health advocate, Ann Wigmore found herself confronting a colon cancer diagnosis at age 50. She embarked upon a course of eating raw greens, blended seeds and grains. She was cancer free within a year. She explored the many raw greens, seeds and grains and believe that wheatgrass had the most powerful healing properties. Proponents of her approach believe that wheatgrass juice has powerful healing and cleansing properties and provides significant alkaline benefits.[13]

Wheatgrass Nutrition

Wheatgrass juice contains 13 vitamins, antioxidants, minerals and trace elements. It's also packed with life-giving enzymes and is highly alkaline, making it perfect for those seeking to eat an alkaline diet.[14]

The antioxidants in wheat grass juice are particularly interesting. Superoxide dismutase, or SOD for short, is a potent antioxidant found in wheatgrass juice and many other plants that battles superoxide, the most harmful free radical in the body. SOD also acts as an anti-inflammatory agent.

Many, many other antioxidants are found in abundance in wheatgrass juice.

How to Enjoy Wheatgrass

Some people grow their own wheatgrass. Others purchase juice at juice bars or have it added to freshly juiced beverages. If you choose to grow your own wheatgrass, many people insist that it must be juiced immediately after cutting. Some research shows that you can get the same high quality juice preparing it within four hours of cutting.

You can drink wheatgrass juice straight, or blend it with other juices. Some people new to wheatgrass juice find it is too powerful for them, especially if they have consumed the Standard American Diet (SAD) full of white flour, sugar and other toxic junk. Go slowly with wheatgrass juice if you experience any tummy upset after your first go with it.

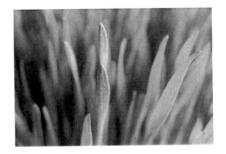

Sprouts

Sprouts are a miracle of nature. Each seed contains the vital essences necessary to create new life. Seeds found in ancient Egyptian tombs can be sprouted. Seeds package all the nutrients a young plant needs to grow into one miniscule container.

One of the most beneficial foods anyone can eat on an alkaline diet are sprouts. If eating sprouts conjures images of hippies in Birkenstocks munching on nasty looking sandwiches, think again. Sprouts have gone mainstream! While sprouting your own seeds at home is easy and economical, you can even buy sprouts at major supermarkets like Wal-Mart, Kroger and Stop & Shop.

Health Benefits of Eating Sprouts

Sprouts have long been touted as an excellent source of vitamins, minerals, phytochemicals and enzymes. But new research sheds light on some of the more powerful health benefits of eating sprouts.

According to Sprout Net[15], studies on alfalfa sprouts indicate that it is high in canavanine, an amino acid analog. Canavanine has demonstrated benefits against pancreatic and colon cancer, as well as leukemia. Other types of sprouts provide different health benefits:

• Alfalfa sprouts: contains amino acids that may fight colon and pancreatic cancer, as well as leukemia. Also rich in saponins, a compound that stimulates the immune system. The immune system is the warrior system of the body that guards against invaders and protects us from viruses, bacteria, and other things that make us sick. Saponins also lower LDL, the so-called "bad cholesterol", without lowering HDL, the "good cholesterol."

- All sprouts contain high amounts of antioxidants. These can protect us against conditions though to contribute to cancer.
- Sprouts also contain plant estrogens that can help women through menopause naturally and safely and prevent bone loss.

So here's to eating more sprouts, both to create an alkaline condition and to contribute to your overall health.

How to Grow Sprouts

Sprouts may seem like magic, but growing them requires no hocus-pocus. All you need to grow sprouts are:

- Sprouts – buy only those seeds marked for sprouting. Purchase them at a health food store, natural health store, or online. Do not try to sprout packets of seeds bought at a garden center! Many are treated with chemicals to keep them suitable for planting, and you don't want to eat those. Try alfalfa sprouts, sunflower sprouts, lentils, mung beans, broccoli, radish and many other tasty sprouts.
- Clean Container – you can buy a sprouting kit, which will include a container and lid or a tray and lid. Or just wash and rinse thoroughly any container you have at hand. You can use recycled glass containers, such

as those used for condiments, jams or jelly. Just be sure to wash them so that no trace of the original food remains, rinse thoroughly, and dry.

- Stockings or Cheesecloth – an old pair of panty hose can be cut up and use to make a screen for the top of your sprouting jar. You can also use cheesecloth, but some people find it expensive. You'll need a screen of some sort. It doesn't have to be perfect. You just need cloth that will allow air to circulate and make it easy for your to drain off the water.
- Water

To grow your sprouts, follow these steps:

1. Clean your sprouting container thoroughly.
2. Add seeds to the container – start with only about a table

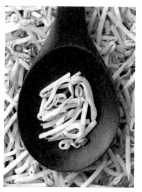

spoon until you get the hang of it. It's better to grow a few sprouts every few days than to grow massive quantities at once and have trouble eating them before they spoil. Start small.
3. Add water to cover the seeds.
4. Cover the top of the jar with your screen of cheesecloth or old stocking. Use a rubber band to affix it to the mouth of the jar.
5. Place the jar somewhere where you can see it. A pantry is fine, or on the kitchen counter.

6. After about 12 hours, drain the water away. Rinse.
7. Rinse the sprouts twice a day. Drain Thoroughly.
8. Within a day or two for some seeds (a bit longer for beans and others), you'll see fresh sprouts. Eat them when they are a few centimeters long. To harvest them, just reach in and grab them!
9. Once fully grown, keep refrigerated.

How to Enjoy Sprouts

There are so many ways to enjoy fresh sprouts. Do eat them fresh, because it is at this time that they are just filled with vibrant enzymes and at their best nutritionally-speaking. You can store them for a day or two in the refrigerator.

Try sprouts in:

- Salads: A natural for sprouts. Grab a big bowl, fill it with greens such as lettuce and spinach, add your favorite vegetables, and top it off with fresh sprouts. Dress it with a little olive oil and balsamic vinegar. Delicious!
- Soups: Mix sprouts into soups for added vegetable power.
- Smoothies: Sprouts blend well into a variety of green smoothies. Just add them when you blend up the vegetables.
- Sandwiches and wraps: Pack sprouts onto tuna fish salad sandwiches, grilled vegetable sandwiches, and other delicious wraps. They add crunch, fiber, and zing to any lunch.
- Other dishes: You can add sprouts wherever you add vegetables. Experiment a bit to accommodate your taste.

Vegetarian, Vegan and Raw Food Lifestyle: Anti Cancer and Health Promoting

As you can see, most research points to the consumption of meat, dairy, and processed foods in the link between cancer and diet. Each of these foods is difficult to digest and deposits toxins in the body. They also contribute to an acidic condition in the body, which we'll talk more about in a later section. What you need to know now is that acidic conditions contribute to cancer formation, while alkaline conditions decrease the likelihood.

Between the high fat, lack of fiber, heavy dose of hormones and antibiotics, and the many other problems associated with eating animal flesh, it's no wonder that more and more people are turning to the Vegetarian, Vegan and raw Vegan diets for health and well-being.

Vegetarian and Vegan: What is the Difference?

Most people know that Vegetarians do not eat meat. Many people think that the terms Vegetarian and Vegan are synonymous, but there are some key differences. Vegetarians may eat products made by animals, such as milk, eggs, cheese, butter, and even honey. They do not eat the flesh of mammals, birds or fish.

Vegans on the other hand do not consume any animal flesh or products. They do not use eggs, cheese, butter or milk, nor will they eat fish.

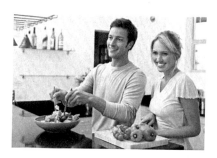

Some Vegans take their dietary choices a step further and embrace what is called a raw or living food diet. These people believe that eating food as close to its natural state as possible—uncooked, fresh, and unprocessed— is the most healthful way of eating. Mimicking the diet of our nearest mammalian relatives, the great apes and chimps, they strive to make vegetables the

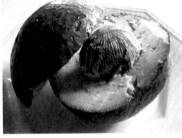

bulk of their diet, laced with fresh fruit, nuts, seeds, and oils, in any combination. Foods are never heated above 116 degrees. Raw Food followers believe that cooking foods destroys the enzymes in the foods.

A Raw Food diet isn't for everyone. Some may find the diet too difficult to follow and too restrictive. Easing gradually into a healthier diet, by decreasing white sugar, flour, caffeine and alcohol and increasing healthy and good-for-you fruits, vegetables and whole grains is something most health experts agree can improve health. If you have any medical conditions, consult your physician or healthcare practitioner before

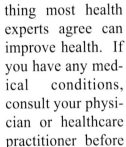

embarking on any diet program such as a raw food diet .

Enzymes[16] are chemicals that facilitate and accelerate chemical reactions in the body. Everyone is born with enzymes and the body takes in new enzymes every time you eat a piece of uncooked fruit or a vegetable. Without enzymes, the chemical reactions that take place every second of the day as part of our natural metabolic processes would stop.

Some Raw Food diet followers believe that we use up certain enzymes, especially given that most people are exposed to a great deal of toxins in the environment, and the typical American diet uses up a lot more enzymes to digest the food than are contributed by the food itself.

Whether or not this is true, its impact on health and cancer formation remains to be proven by scientific research. What we do know is that enzymes are vital for health and well-being, and fresh fruits and vegetables contain them in abundance.

A raw and living foods diet can be a wonderful, life-affirming diet, but it's not for everyone. Changing to a raw food diet takes time and patience. It definitely supports an anti-cancer philosophy and lifestyle since a raw diet excludes meat, dairy, alcohol, and caffeine, and includes an abundance of fiber, vitamins, minerals and phytochemicals from all the wonderful, rich plant-based sources found in the diet.

For more information on a raw and living food diet, visit Raw People (www.RawPeople.com).

Chapter Two
The Acid-Alkaline Connection

By now, we hope we have presented enough information and facts that you are ready to take charge of your health and embrace a diet based on whole foods as a cancer preventative measure. Diet is an important milestone in the fight against cancer. The abundance of phytochemicals in fresh fruits, vegetables and whole grains provides the body with the chemical substances it needs to fight cancerous conditions on the cellular level. Fiber mechanically speeds along waste products and toxins that need to be expelled through the body so that they can't stick to the intestinal walls and damage the cells or reabsorb back into the body. Enzymes, which help facilitate chemical processes, contribute to our health and well-being with each apple we munch or celery stick we crunch. Phytochemicals in the ruby red grapefruit and royal purple grape battle DNA changes, while other chemicals fight bacteria and more.

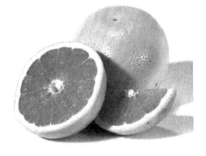

But there's more to fresh fruits and vegetables than this wonderful symphony of chemical reactions. A delicate balancing act is played out with every breath you take and every sip of water. It's the acid-alkaline balance.

Acid, Alkaline, and Neutral

Foods		pH	Substances
Pork, Veal, Hamburgers, Polished White Rice	Acid	pH=0	Battery Acid, Strong Hydrochloic Acid
Beef Oysters, Crab, Lobster, Shrimp		pH=1	Hydrochloic Acid Secreated by Stomach Lining
Ham, Turkey, Chicken, Coffee, Tea		pH=2	Lemon Juice, Gastric Acid, Vinagar
Eggs, Liqour, Chocolate		pH=3	Grapefruit Juice, Orange Juice, Soda
Hard Cheese (Parmesan), Fish		pH=4	Acid Rain, Tomatoe Juice, Beer
Brown & Wild Rice, Beer, Wine			
Most Breads, Pasta, Spaghetti			
Whole Grain Breads, Magarine, Nuts		pH=5	Soft Drinking Water, Black Coffee, Pure Rain
Butter & Cream, Soft Cheeses		pH=6	Urine, Saliva, Egg Yolks, Cow's Milk
Whey, Cow's & Goats Milk	Neutral 7.35-7.45	pH=7	Pure Water
Potatoes, Lentils, Onions, Garlic		pH=8	Sea Water
Apples, Pears, Bananas, Oranges		pH=9	Baking Soda
Olives, Molasses, Cabbage, Lettuce			
Dandelon Greens, Soy Nuts		pH=10	Great Salt Lake, Milk of Magnesia, Detergent
Beets, Celery, Carrots, Tomatoes		pH=11	Ammonia Solution, Household Cleaners
Dried Figs, Mushrooms		pH=12	Soapy Water
Pure Lecithin, Ginger, Spinach		pH=13	Bleaches, Oven Cleaner, Household Lye
Cucumbers, Radishes, Squash	Base	pH=14	Liquid Drain Cleaner

Although we hate to do this to you, we're going to revisit your high school chemistry class.

If you can think back to that time, try to picture the pH scale. It's a scale from 0 to 14 that measures how acidic or alkaline a substance is based on various tests. A pH level of 7 is considered neutral—right in the middle of the scale. The high end of the scale is considered alkaline.

Why is it important to understand the pH scale and what each of these terms mean? Living creatures usually thrive somewhere near the middle or balanced part of the pH scale, with some exceptions (certain bacteria, for example, can live in the extremely acidic conditions of the stomach and cause stomach ulcers). The human body is a complex yet delicate system, and it must maintain a pH of 7.4 for optimal health.

Note that the pH of 7.4 is the overall pH; some parts of the body may be more acidic. The stomach, for example, is acidic because food must be digested. Blood pH must be a steady 7.35 to 7.45; if it falls below or rises above, serious illness or death can result.

Homeostasis, Or Keeping Things Balanced

Think for a moment about what's going on inside your body right now, as you're sitting reading these words. Your brain is busy processing the information, neurons firing, some storing the information. Your eyes are tracking the words, sending signals to the brain. Your heart beats, sending blood whooshing throughout the system, while the kidneys filter the blood. The stomach, small and large intestines are busy digesting your lunch. At the cellular level, hundreds of processes are going on all at once. Cells are dividing, dying, absorbing nutrients, reporting invaders and calling for the white blood cell army.

Within all of this, a chorus of chemical messengers must sing in tune to keep all processes harmonious. To do their job efficiently, they must have the right chemical components, including the proper pH.

How Acidity Affects the Body

What happens when one singer in the chorus goes off key? It can throw off the entire work. This is also true with the body.

Every food has a different pH. Some foods are highly acidic, like meat, milk and white sugar, while other foods are alkaline. Water out of the tap is usually neutral, but depending on where you live, it may vary from slightly acidic to slightly alkaline. True alkaline mineral water, created by special machines, creates water with varying alkaline pH levels.

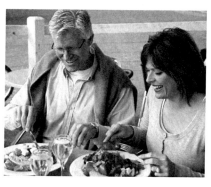

Let's imagine a typical lunch. Today's lunch, purchased from the deli, will include a ham sandwich on white bread, a bag of potato chips, and a can of cola soda pop. This is a very normal

American lunch and a highly acidic lunch. On the typical scale of foods, processed flour (made into white bread) is extremely acidic, while pork or ham products come a close second. Potatoes are alkaline, but frying them in oil and salting them to make potato chips makes them more acidic. Soda pop's white sugar is acidic enough without adding phosphoric acid to it—the typical ingredient in cola—which is acid indeed!

So, you eat your ham sandwich, munch your chips, and wash it down with pop. You then return to work. Your stomach accepts the contents, and the acids begin to digest them. The pH of what leaves the stomach is going to be low—very acidic. As the acidic mix moves through the diges-tive system, the body strives to return to homeostasis, or balance. It will need to rebalance the pH. How does it do that?

Think back again to high school chemistry class. A buffer solu-tion is one that neutralizes acid or weakens it. The body, in its infinite wisdom, seeks to buffer the acids from that lunch sand-wich and cola. How does it do that? It seeks minerals, such as calcium and magnesium, to buf-fer the acids. If the minerals are available in the foods, it will use those first. If not, it begins to scavenge them from around the body. Thus, drinking soda pop, a highly acidic beverage, not only bathes teeth in an acidic solution full of sugar that encourages the bacteria the causes tooth decay, it rots teeth from the inside out, because the body will leach calcium right from the teeth to buffer the acids, along with calcium from the skeleton.

Does this sound crazy? Listen to what two professors of medical research and clinical nutrition, Deanne M. Minich, PhD., and Jeffrey S. Bland, PhD, said:

In the setting of inadequate intake of bicarbonate precursors, buffers in the bone matrix neutralize the excess diet-derived acid, and in the process, bone becomes demineralized. Excess diet-derived acid titrates bone and lead to increased urinary calcium and reduced urinary citrate excretion. The resultant adverse clinical consequences are possibly increased bone demineralized and increased risk of calcium containing kidney stones.[17]

In other words:

- Eating and drinking too many acidic foods and beverages throws the body's acid/alkaline balance off kilter;
- Unless you take in enough bicarbonates (buffers), the body uses minerals in the bones as buffers to rebalance or achieve homeostasis;
- The resulting consequences are 1) demineralized bones and 2) increased calcium citrate excretion in urine;
- The possible diseases resulting from this include osteoporosis, tooth decay, arthritis, and kidney stones;
- Depletion of magnesium as the body uses this vital mineral to buffer excess acids;

So, if you want to be sick, keep eating that ham sandwich and washing it down with soda pop. Although one meal like that won't kill you, a constant diet of primarily acidic foods, eaten over many years, sets the stages for these ailments…or worse.

Protein and Digestive Waste

We've mentioned before that protein foods, namely beef, dairy products, pork and chicken, are highly acidic. The reason is simple: the digestion of protein leads to strong acids in our bodies, like sulfuric acid, phosphoric acid, and nitric acid. According to Dennis Myers, M.D, and Robert Miller, D.C., "These acids are strong, like the battery acid in your car."[18] According to Drs. Myers and Miller, the constant influx of protein and acid-rich foods cause both a toxic build up and an acidic environment.

Keep in mind that the body has to do something with toxins. Whether ingested through the foods we eat or the air we breathe, toxins are either excreted through urine, feces, breath or perspiration, or they are stored—usually in the fatty tissues of the body. The body puts a protective coating of fat around them to keep the harmful elements away from the vital organs. This is one of the reasons people put on excess weight.

Robert O. Young, PhD and author of the book, The pH Miracle for Weight Loss, demonstrates this effectively in the book through photographs of blood samples. When patients ate protein-rich foods like bacon and eggs, there is a marked and unhealthy difference in their blood samples than patients on an alkaline-rich diet. You can learn more about this on his website, http://www.phmiracleliving.com

Acidity and Cancer

So between the buildup of toxins from eating the wrong foods and the chronic acidic condition in the body from years of ingesting processed, acid-rich foods, it's no wonder that cancer is an epidemic in industrialized societies. Think about the diets of indigenous people; while cancer isn't unheard of, it's rare. Consider the diets of indigenous people. Westin Price, DDS, a researcher, traveled the world in the early 1930s and studied the diets of the last remaining pockets of society that did not eat a so-called modern diet. From the rugged Hebrides Islands of Scotland to remote mountain valleys in Switzerland, he recorded through notes, photographs, and dental records (he was a dentist and former president of the American Dental Association) the health and diseases of the people, as well as their diet. No matter what are of the world he visited, from African tribesmen to Swiss mountain villages, he observed that the native cultural diet, typically rich in plants and grains, resulted in hardy, healthy people with little tooth decay. Once the 'modern' diet filled with sugar and white flour came into their lives, the people's health rapidly deteriorated. And while Dr. Price did not make the connected between the acidic nature of white sugar and flour, we now know that these foods, in addition to being harder to digest and lacking many vitamins and minerals, also create acidic conditions in the body.

One of the most compelling studies demonstrating how an acidic condition in cells encourages the formation of cancer was conducted over 75 years ago. Dr. Otto

Warburg won a Nobel Prize for this research. Dr. Warburg demonstrated that a lack of oxygen to cells made them revert to another method of obtaining energy, resulting in a buildup of lactic acid. The acidic conditions result in uncontrolled replication of the DNA and RNA in the cell nucleus, and the formation of cancer.[19]

Other studies over time have also demonstrated that acidic conditions damage the cell's control center, resulting in out of control cell division. Alkaline conditions, on the other hand, appear to encourage healthy cells.

The Alkaline Diet and Cancer Prevention

To sum up everything that we've said so far:

- There is a correlation between diet and cancer, especially certain cancers.
- Many factors contribute to cancer. There is no one cause. Interplay among diet, heredity, mental stress, and environment are all thought to contribute to the development of cancer.
- Diet is within the control of the individual.
- Certain diets are believed to decrease the likelihood of cancer, as evidenced by many well-known studies in both conventional and alternative medicine.

- As early as the 1930s, doctors and researchers knew that acidic conditions encouraged uncontrolled cell growth, but mainstream physicians believe that the body pH is always set…that what you eat doesn't change that.

But what if you could take charge of your health…and eat to ward off cancer?

An alkaline diet is the key. Full of healthy vegetables, fruits and grains, and ionized alkaline mineral water, an alkaline diet supports cancer prevention by:

- Increasing the intake of alkaline-forming foods, and decreasing or eliminating acidic foods;
- Increasing fiber intake, which is important in the prevention of many types of cancer;
- Increasing the level of anti-oxidants, found in abundance in fruits, vegetables and grains, and known for their ability to mop up free radicals which can damage cellular DNA and set the stage for cancer growth;
- Decreasing your fat intake, since a plant-based diet is naturally low in fat, especially harmful saturated fats.

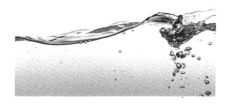

But These Foods Taste Acidic to Me!

One of the most puzzling things for people new to an alkaline diet and lifestyle is that many foods that appear on the list of alkaline foods taste acidic. Some people even say that the foods give them acidic indigestion! Let's tackle both of these reactions.

Foods that Taste Acidic… but are Alkaline

The pH of a food is not measured in taste. It's not even measured when the food is in its original state. A new method called the PRAL score is used to measure the acidity of foods.

According to Dr. Peter Kopko, D.C. :

In 1995 two researchers, Dr. Thomas Remer and Dr. F. Manz, developed a new way to measure the acid/base effect of specific foods on the human body. This pH measuring tool is referred to as the Potential Renal Acid Load (**PRAL**). The PRAL of an ingested specific food is determined by measuring the acidity and ammonium appearing in the urine and then subtracting out the measured urinary bicarbonate. This method yields a net acid excretion score based on direct measurements of the urine. Previous to the imple mentation of the PRAL score method ash analysis was utilized.

The PRAL method is far superior to ash analysis in that

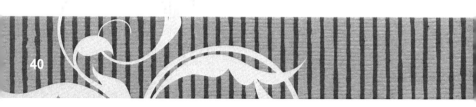

it takes into effect the digestion and absorption of a food and its direct effect on the kidneys and urine. However in my opinion the PRAL method has some limitations as well in that a specific food may elicit a pH homeostatic balancing mechanism and that would influence the end result in the urine. This may be evidenced by the PRAL score of coffee (listed as alkaline). Nevertheless, the PRAL method remains the best method to date.[20]

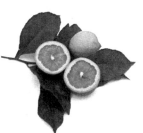

The bottom line is that taste doesn't tell you much about the acid or alkaline nature of the foods you're eating. So pucker up. Citrus fruits can be alkaline!

Acid Indigestion

Many people claim that eating the foods on the alkaline diet recommended here give them indigestion. "I can't eat peppers," they'll say. "I get acid indigestion."

People experience acid indigestion as a painful burning feeling in the abdomen or stomach area. While it may indeed be caused by eating a food rich in acids, it can also be caused by not having enough stomach acids. Many people who have acid reflux disease, for example, take antacids, only to find that they don't help. That's because antacids neutralize acid, and the problem isn't too much acid—it's either a mechanical problem (trouble with the flap on top of the stomach not closing properly, thus regurgitating acid) or their stomachs actually lack enough acids to process the foods adequately. An alkaline, plant-based diet and alkaline water can help this condition.

**The Alkaline Diet:
What to Eat to Prevent Cancer**

The alkaline diet is simple, natural, and healthful. It provides abundant fiber, vitamins, minerals, carbohydrates, proteins, and fats. The emphasis is on fresh, wholesome, natural fruits, vegetables and grains, monosaturated plant-based oils, and as much raw, uncooked foods as you can eat.

Two of the very best foods you can eat to alkalize the body are

sprouts of all kinds and wheat grass juice. Raisins are also extremely alkalizing, and many alternative health professionals recommend eating a handful of raisins each day to alkalize the body.

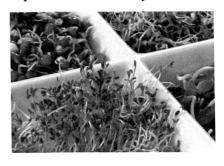

In this diet, you'll emphasize:

Vegetables: From legumes to lettuce, you can eat an abundance of healthy vegetables. The accompanying chart will show you which vegetable to choose from among the most alkalizing vegetables.

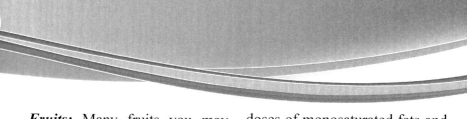

Fruits: Many fruits you may imagine to be acidic are actually alkaline. Grapefruit, for example, tastes acidic but is actually an alkalizing fruit. Follow the suggestions on the chart to ensure the most alkalizing effect.

Grains: Grains and cereals tend to be acidic, so eat sparingly or the lowest alkaline on the list. The best choices include oats, quinoa, and wild rice.

Seeds: Many seeds taste delicious, are portable and good for snacking, and they're alkalizing. Pumpkin seeds are highly alkalizing.

Oils: The healthiest oils to include are vegetable oils, like sesame seed oil, coconut oil, flax oil and olive oil. Not only do they provide heart-healthy doses of monosaturated fats and omega fatty acids, they are also alkalizing rather than acidifying.

Meat and Dairy: Sadly for you carnivores out there, but for the best cancer-prevention efforts, meats should be eliminated. Many studies cited here and even more published in reputable medical journals point to a correlation between high beef diets and high cancer rates. Whether it's the intense acidic nature of the meat or the high fat content remains to be verified, but for those seeking an alkaline diet, meat is best left off the plate and the shopping cart altogether.

Dairy is also surprisingly acidic. Many dairy foods are also combined with white sugar, another very acidic food. Ice cream, unfortunately, is not an anti-cancer food and is at the ultimate end of the acid scale. If you're an ice cream fanatic, don't panic; there are some health alternatives for frozen treats made with fruit that you'll swear taste like your favorite Baskin-Robbins. We promise!

Beverages

By far the best beverage you can consume is water. Our bodies contain a tremendous amount of water. It's used in nearly every metabolic process. We can live without food for several days or weeks, but without water we die very quickly.

Many people are walking around in a state of constant dehydration. They believe

they are well hydrated as they guzzle diet sodas or coffee, but the fact of the matter is that much of the liquid they ingest is excreted, thanks to the witches' brew of caffeine and chemicals in the beverage. Plus, more water may be lost as the body fights to rid itself of these unsavory characters.

Although fruit juices, especially fresh squeezed or pressed fruit and vegetable juices, are a healthy option, water quenches the thirst, supports health, and is calorie-free.

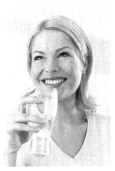

If you've never tried alkaline water, it may be worth investing. The next chapter will delve more deeply into the benefits of alkaline water and how this helps with cancer prevention. Ionized

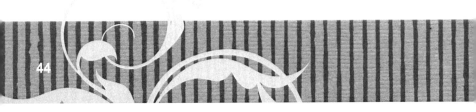

alkaline water is tap water that is run through a special machine and through electrolysis, it raises the pH. The high pH water is alkaline mineral water for drinking and the lower pH byproduct is called acid water. It can be used for bathing and washing dishes and can kill bacteria effectively. In fact it's so effective that acid water is used in some hospitals around the world to disinfect surgical tools.

Ionized alkaline mineral water is one of the best ways you can raise your pH. Even if you choose not to drink ionized alkaline water, do switch from your current beverages to plain, healthy spring water. You can easily sabotage your alkaline diet efforts by washing down that big salad with gallons of soda pop and coffee.

Just a quick note here about water from reverse osmosis filters and bottled water. While both may be better for you than city tap water, unfortunately they don't confer the same benefits as ionized alkaline water. Reverse osmosis actually produces water that is acidic. Bottled water is, frankly, no better than tap water, and most are acidic. For a complete list of acidic bottle waters, see the book The *pH Miracle for Weight Loss* by Dr. Robert O. Young in the Resources section.

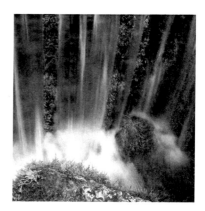

The Top Ten Cancer Fighting Foods

Studies have shown that the following ten foods are the best at beating cancer. According to the National Cancer Institute, "Diets rich in fruits and vegetables may reduce the risk of certain types of cancer and chronic disease." According to the Diet Channel[21], here are the top ten cancer fighting foods:

1. Tomatoes
2. Broccoli Sprouts
3. Berries
4. Soybeans
5. Tea
6. Pumpkin
7. Spinach
8. Garlic
9. Pineapple
10. Apple

Food Preparation

Cooking techniques are also important on an alkaline, cancer-preventing diet. You've probably heard or read that frying foods is bad for you. It's the worst cooking method you can choose if cancer is a concern. Deep fat frying, like fast food restaurants use to cook potatoes into French fries, adds carcinogens to the food. It also intensely acidifies them. Avoid fried foods. Most doctors, from naturopaths to conventional physicians, will agree on this point.

What most people don't realize, however, is that cooking—no matter how benign— actually acidifies foods to some degrees. So, the more raw, uncooked foods you can eat, the better. A diet consisting of nothing but raw foods is called a raw, Vegan, or living diet. Yes, it's possible to eat a satisfying, healthy diet on nothing but uncooked foods. We'll go more into this dietary choice later. Know right now that eating nothing but raw foods is probably one of the healthier cancer-fighting things you can do.

If you must cook your food, steaming or baking is preferable. Some people believe that microwaving foods is harmful. The jury is still out on this. If you're concerned about the potential consequences of microwaving food, steaming is easy and just about as quick.

What to Eat on an Alkaline Diet?

Focus on Fruit: Berries

Christine Sardo, the person managing the clinical trials on berry consumption and cancer prevention at Ohio State University's College of Medicine, stated at a conference in 2006 that, "We are promoting the concept of 'fruitraceuticals' as opposed to pharmaceuticals for cancer, and emphasizing prevention vs. treatment." Berries, from the common strawberry to the exotic acai berry from South America, are proving to be potent cancer fighters. These sweet, delicious treats contain an abundance of cancer-fighting compounds, including antioxidants. Studies published in the journal Cancer Research demonstrate that rats that eat berries had a large reduction in various cancers, as compared to rats that didn't eat the berries.[22] These findings are exciting, especially because berries taste good! Fill up your plate with a rainbow of berries: raspberries, blackberries, strawberries, cranberries, blueberries, and any other berry available to you. With just 46 calories for a one cup serving of strawberries and more than the RDA for vitamin C alone, berries are a wonderfully delicious cancer-fighting food.

ALKALINE FOODS

VEGETABLES

Asparagus
Artichokes
Cabbage
Lettuce
Onion
Cauliflower
Radish
Swede
Lambs Lettuce
Peas
Courgette
Red Cabbage
Leeks
Watercress
Spinach
Turnip
Chives
Carrot
Green Beans
Beetroot
Garlic
Celery
Grasses (wheat, straw, barley, dog, kamut etc.)
Cucumber
Broccoli
Kale
Brussels Sprouts

FRUITS

Lemon
Lime
Avocado
Tomato
Grapefruit
Watermelon (is neutral)
Rhubarb

DRINKS

'Green Drinks'
Fresh vegetable juice
Pure water (**distilled** or **ionized**)
Lemon water (pure water + fresh lemon or lime).
Herbal Tea
Vegetable broth
Non-sweetened Soy Milk
Almond Milk

SEEDS, NUTS & GRAINS

Almonds
Pumpkin
Sunflower
Sesame
Flax
Buckwheat Groats
Spelt
Lentils
Cumin Seeds
Any sprouted seed

FATS & OILS

Flax
Hemp
Avocado
Olive
Evening Primrose
Borage
Coconut Oil
Oil Blends (such as **Udo's Choice**)

OTHERS

Sprouts (soy, alfalfa, mung bean, wheat, little radish , chickpea, broccoli etc)
Bragg Liquid Aminos (Soy Sauce Alternative)
Hummus
Tahini

ACIDIC FOODS	
MEATS Pork Lamb Beef Chicken Turkey Crustaceans Other Seafood (apart from occasional oily fish such as salmon)	**DAIRY PRODUCTS** Milk Eggs Cheese Cream Yogurt Ice Cream
OTHERS Vinegar White Pasta White Bread Wholemeal Bread Biscuits Soy Sauce Tamari Condiments (Tomato Sauce, Mayonnaise etc.) Artificial Sweeteners Honey	**DRINKS** Fizzy Drinks Coffee Tea Beers Spirits Fruit Juice Dairy Smoothies Milk Traditional Tea
CONVENIENCE FOODS Sweets Chocolate Microwave Meals Tinned Foods Powdered Soups Instant Meals Fast Food	**FATS & OILS** Saturated Fats Hydrogenated Oils Margarine (worse than Butter) Corn Oil Vegetable Oil Sunflower Oil
FRUITS All fruits aside from those listed in the alkaline column.	**SEEDS & NUTS** Peanuts Cashew Nuts Pistachio Nut

Transitioning to an Alkaline Diet

The simplest way to begin eating an alkaline diet is to transition gradually. You can do this by:

1. Eliminate the white: This means anything pure white should go from the diet. White sugar, white flour, white bread and crackers, and milk should be removed immediately. These are all highly acidic foods.
2. Eliminate caffeine and alcohol. While tea is a powerful cancer-fighting beverage, you're better off with plain water or alkaline water to fight cancer.
3. Reducing or eliminating dairy products. If you're concerned about getting enough calcium, eat more green leafy vegetables. These contain an abundance of minerals, including calcium. Exercise also improves bone density, especially weight training, so you can continue to build strong bones without excessive calcium consumption.
4. Reduce or eliminate meat, poultry and fish. Start with the obvious bad guys: luncheon meats and hot dogs filled with meat "by products," nitrates and preservatives. Then eliminate beef, pork, poultry and fish in that order. Many people worry about consuming adequate protein without eating meat or dairy. The latest findings indicate that the diet should be no more than 20% protein[23]; most people can get plenty of healthy protein from vegetables. Do you think that all of those muscular football players you see in the NFL eat steaks all day? Many of them are Vegetarians and even Vegans, consuming no animal

products whatsoever. If you eat a healthy diet rich in alkaline foods, you should be in no danger of too little protein.

5. Increase fruit and vegetable consumption.

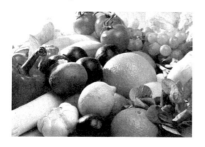

A Sample Menu

Most doctors recommend that alkaline diets contain 75% highly alkaline food, and the remaining 25% can lean towards acidic. Try to consume approximately 75% of your foods as raw or lightly cooked fruits and vegetables, with the remaining 25% grains, grain products, oils, nuts and seeds.

If you decide to continue eating some meat, a little poultry or fish can be taken in that 25% of your total food intake.

Here's what a sample day's menu on the alkaline diet will look like:

Breakfast

- Large fruit salad OR
- Alkaline granola or raw granola, made with raw nuts, seeds, berries and taken with almond milk OR
- Green smoothie, made of blended fruits and greens OR
- Fruit only smoothie, blended fruits

Snack

- Fruit of your choice

Lunch

- Large salad of mixed greens, topped with dressing made of olive oil, lemon juice and sea salt OR
- Lentil soup with lightly steamed vegetables OR Vegetable soup with whole grain bread (not white bread) OR
- Tuna salad made with tuna, celery, onions and dressed with olive oil only, served over bed of leafy green vegetables OR
- Stuffed baked potato—baked potato stuffed with steamed broccoli, cauliflower, peppers, carrots and vegetables of your choice, drizzled with olive oil and lightly sprinkled with sea salt

Snack

- Green smoothie OR
- Fruit of your choice OR
- Carrot, celery, broccoli, cauliflower and other vegetables, cut into chunks and dressed with a little sprinkle of salt and pepper

Dinner

- Pasta, made from buckwheat, rice, amaranth or quinoa, topped with broccoli rabe or Swiss Chard lightly sautéed in olive oil and garlic, with a side dish of steamed vegetables OR
- 3 oz poultry or fish, with two vegetables of your choice

If you're still hungry, add a big salad.

For dessert, choose from the abundance of wholesome fruits

available in season. Some raw food recipes make wonderful alkaline diet desserts, such as raw cheesecake, raw chocolates, etc. Look the ingredients list over carefully and match it to the low alkaline foods.

Remember that this is only a sample menu. If you look over the choices of acid and alkaline foods on the chart,

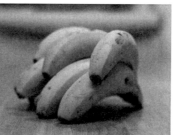

choose from the alkaline side, mix and match the foods, and create a variety of meals of your choice. Remember that variety ensures adequate nutritional intake, so the more variety you can work into the diet, the better.

Treats

Giving up sweet treats is often the hardest part of changing to an alkaline diet. Ice cream is one of the most acidic foods, so it should be eliminated from the diet. But you can make an ice cream like treat that has the coldness, sweetness, and consistency of your favorite treat.

Here's how:

Run frozen peeled bananas and/or coconut meat and almond milk through your juicer. Remember to peel the bananas first, before freezing them. It will taste like soft serve ice cream. If you don't own a juicer, try mashing the bananas and freezing them. You can also freeze unsweetened fruit juice or green smoothies into popsicle forms to enjoy the quintessential summer treat without any added sugar or chemical colors and flavors. Yum!

Raw and Vegan Foods

Some people take this diet a step further and embark on what is called either a raw food diet or a living foods diet. The concept is simple: that heating foods above 118 degrees Fahrenheit destroys vital enzymes. Raw food diet followers make delicious meals and dishes from raw, unprocessed and uncooked foods. If this sounds appealing, there's a lot of information available online to get you started. Raw People (www.RawPeople.com) is a great resource for those starting out on a raw and Vegan diet and has many recipes available.

The Anti Cancer Diet: Good Health Through Foods

"Let food be your medicine." While scientists don't understand all the causes for every type of cancer, we do know that lifestyle choices contribute to the formation of various types of cancers. So let your food be your medicine and choose healthy, alkaline forming foods as the basis of your diet.

CHAPTER 3
What You Need to Know About Water

Throughout this book, we've mentioned alkaline mineral water a few times, so we'd like to take a moment now and tell you a bit more about alkaline water and how it works with an alkaline diet to fight the formation of cancer. These statements haven't been studied by the FDA, but many people do believe that alkaline mineral water can contribute to a healthy lifestyle. This short chapter will give you an introduction

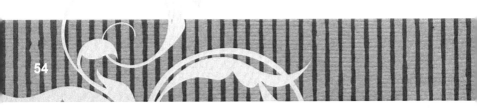

to ionized alkaline mineral water and its place in an alkaline diet. For more information, visit the website, www.LifeIonizers.com.

What is Alkaline Ionized Water?

Alkaline water is common tap water that has been run through a special machine that separates the molecules into two streams, one acidic, the other alkaline. Ionized alkaline water has a pH of 7 –10+, but many alkaline water machines have an adjustment that lets you set the pH of the water. You drink the

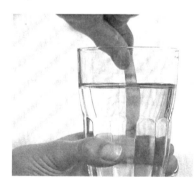

ionized alkaline water and use the acidic water for cleaning. Acidic water is an excellent sanitizing agent, and can be used around the house for everything from cleaning cutting boards after preparing foods to washing dishes.

The Difference Between Alkaline Water Ionizers and Water Purifiers

Many of you reading this right now may be a little puzzled. Glancing at the kitchen faucet, you may wonder, "But I have a filter and use one of those filtration pitcher things. Isn't my water good for me?" Yes and no. Clearly, drinking filtered water is better than guzzling diet soda, but alkaline water is very different from purified water.

Water purifiers do not alter the pH of the water itself, nor do they change the makeup of the water. Rather, they filter, or remove, off tastes, chemicals, and sometimes minerals. Most of these systems use charcoal or some other filtration method to screen out the harmful elements in water. The resulting water may look clearer and taste better, but it has not been fundamentally altered.

Ionized alkaline mineral water is different. When it passes through an alkaline water ionizer, it goes through the process of electrolysis. The process of ionization gives the water its special properties. After it filters the water and then passes it through an electrolysis chamber, it splits the water into two streams. One stream is alkaline minerals for drinking and the other is acidic minerals for sanitizing. When you look at water molecules under a microscope, the molecules form clusters of about 13 molecules or more. Ionized, alkaline water clusters are smaller, typically just 6 molecules in a cluster and have a negative charge. This difference is important. It helps the body use the clusters more efficiently, and hydrates more effectively. This negatively charged, micro-clustered water also helps detoxify at the cellular level by combining with the positive ions of heavy metals and other contaminants and then flushes them out of the cells. Since the alkaline minerals are concentrated, this water helps the body create a more balanced pH. Most people on a standard Western diet have a urine pH in the range of 4.5-5.9, which is very acidic. Remember that pH is measured with a logarithmic scale, just like earthquakes. This means if your urine pH is 5.0 and if your goal was 7.0, your urine is 100 times too acidic. Most people with cancer tend to have very acidic urine. This type of water can help balance the body's pH, hydrate more efficiently, detoxify the cells and deliver nutrients more effectively.

What about reverse-osmosis filtration systems? The problem again with reverse-osmosis filtration system is that they are simply filtration systems. In this system, water is forced through a membrane-like filter with tiny holes in it. Most heavy metals and contaminants are removed in this method. However, the water is acidic—the pH is below 7, usually in the mid 6 range. If you believe that alkaline, rather than acidic, water leads to good health, then it makes sense that a reverse-osmosis filtration system does nothing good for health and can simply add to the acidic balance that most people are carrying around with them.[24] That, combined with the fact that reverse osmosis water is deficient in minerals, makes the consumption of this water detrimental to one's health.

Bottled waters may appear on the surface to be a healthier alternative, but would you believe that most bottled waters are actually acidic? It's true. While water typically has a neutral pH of 7, Dr. Robert O. Young[25] tested 60 of the best-known brands of bottled water. His findings indicate that 30 brands have pH levels below 7.0, meaning that they are acidic. According to Dr. Young, 25% of all bottled waters are nothing more than municipal water – that's right, tap water!

Besides, who wants to add all that plastic into the landfills? Trucking water from one place to another (or sending it via railway or even by air or sea) burns fossil fuels and contributes to pollution. Bottled waters are no better for you than tap water. You can just as easily place water into a reusable bottle if you want the convenience of drinking water on the go.

So if you're looking for the best water to drink to alkalize your body, choose ionized alkaline water.

Health Benefits of Ionized Alkaline Water

Throughout this booklet, we've tried to impress upon you the importance of maintaining an alkaline, rather than acidic balance in the body. Remember that our bodies do regulate their internal pH to keep us alive. However, when we dump acidic foods and beverages into our bodies, the process of digestion metabolizes those foods and creates an acidic ash or waste that must be expelled or safely stored. Think about a nuclear reactor. As the reactor burns fuel, the spent rods must be stored, for they are radioactive and dangerous, but no more energy can be released from them to produce the final product, electricity. Thus the dangerous rods are stored in lead containers until such time as they naturally decay. Our bodies do the same thing with the waste products of our acidic lifestyles— only they store the byproducts in fat and pad it with water.

It takes time to change the body's balance from acidic to alkaline. One

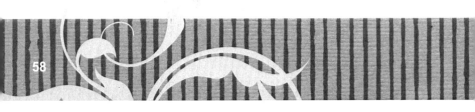

way to hasten this process is to add to your alkaline diet delicious tasting ionized alkaline mineral water.

The health benefits of alkaline water are many and include:

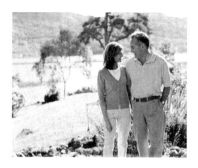

- Improved hydration
- Increased clarity and energy
- Weight loss: time and again, people drinking alkaline water find themselves losing weight. As the acid-alkaline balance shifts and the body moves towards an alkaline state, it releases the stored acidic by products and body fat it used to contain them. Out goes the weight! You can see astonishing before and after photos of people who lost weight after embracing an alkaline lifestyle in the book, *"The pH Miracle For Weight Loss"*, by Robert O. Young.

- Chronic diseases: many people report their symptoms improve when drinking alkaline water. This information is anecdotal, meaning it is not proved by the scientific method or accepted by conventional doctors or the FDA as fact. However, you can find many testimonials from people who claim their diabetes, arthritis, and other inflammatory diseases improved after drinking ionized alkaline mineral water. Remember that Nobel-prize winning scientist from the 1930s we mentioned who discovered that cells like an alkaline condition, but behave erratically and can be damaged by acidic conditions? It is possible that the internal pH, and the body's constant struggle to return to homeostasis, taxes some people, and whether by genetics, environment, or some complex interplay of these various forces, that interaction shows as different diseases. Alkaline water appears to mitigate many of the symptoms associated with chronic diseases as reported by people drinking ionized alkaline mineral water.

Ionized Alkaline Water and Cancer Prevention

According to CancerTutor.com[26], ionized alkaline water acts in three ways to prevent cancer:

1. As an antioxidant, scavenging free radicals before they can damage cell DNA and RNA;
2. It creates an internal alkaline environment, which cancer cells don't like;
3. It provides the body with smaller clusters of water molecules, which helps the water move through the body easier and remove wastes more effectively.

What Research is There on Ionized Alkaline Mineral Water?

Most of the research on ionized water is taking place in Japan and Korea. Some critics of using alkaline water as a preventative or treatment method for cancer scoff at the credentials of these researchers. One chemist even posted a long diatribe against the information because he believes the Koreans and Japanese are more susceptible to what he calls "pseudo-science." These bigoted remarks overlook one fact: that perhaps other scientists are considering different avenues of exploration in the battle against cancer rather than the Western approach of surgery, radiation, and chemotherapy.

Let's face it: despite decades of research, despite improved surgeries and drugs, we are still fumbling around for ways to prevent cancer. And for those in the scientific research community, whose research is often funded by major pharmaceutical companies, what incentive do they have to prevent disease? Shareholders make profits when stocks go up. Drug company stocks go up when they invent new products, i.e., drugs. Drug companies have no vested interest in keeping you healthy. They are committed to relieving diseases, but it is not in their best interest to keep you from getting sick.

If you think the government is interested, think about again. Yes, some money goes towards prevention research. But most money is earmarked with special favors going back to the purveyors of sickness. Most research today is tainted in some way with money from the drug companies, and used with the purpose of fueling drug research. Don't blame the drug companies—that's what they do.

Instead, you must take charge of your health. Whether you choose to believe the many testimonials or claims about ionized alkaline mineral water, or embark on an alkaline diet and lifestyle, that's up to you. But do think about your choices. Don't blindly follow the leader when it comes to your health. Please see the resources section for more information on ionized alkaline mineral water and related topics.

Chapter 4
Other Acidifiers

A long time ago—think *millions of years ago*—our bodies adapted in a very special way to keep us alive. When a saber toothed tiger attacked, our ancestors' bodies flooded with energy. The stomach shut down, adrenaline kicked in, and enough energy surged to help Grandma or Grandpa Cave dweller to fight that tiger or flee from him.

This so-called "fight or flight" mechanism triggers a major acidifier in today's world: stress. But unlike our cave-dwelling ancestors, we typically don't have saber-toothed tigers chasing us through the forest. Instead, we face daily stressors such as:

- Chronic dehydration
- Looming deadlines at work
- Traffic jams
- Fights with bosses, spouse or children
- Tests at school
- Nightly News cast (all gloom and doom, wars and natural disasters)
- Economic insecurity (i.e., fear of losing one's job)
- Emotional turmoil from medical problems, addictions
- Over committing and over scheduling
- Performance (actors, dancers, giving a speech)
- Worry and anxiety
- Dealing with a loved one's illness
- Death of a loved one or pet
- Moving
- Changing jobs
- Getting married
- Getting divorced
- Having a baby
- Adopting children

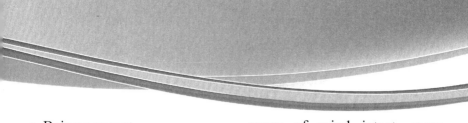

- Being a parent
- Caring for an elderly relative
- Pollution
- Loud noises

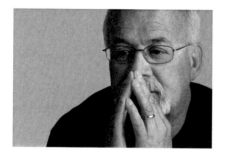

Notice one thing about this list: with the exception of facing severe medical problems, most of these conditions are man-made. Stress is often defined as the feeling one experiences between perceived reality (the stressor) and reality (actuality).

Stress is really in the eye of the beholder. Some people can sail through their day with their peace of mind intact, seeming to let the stresses of the day roll right off their backs. Other people go by the coffee mug saying, "Good morning, let the stress begin." And some stress is actually good for us. There are many science experiments with plants, for example, that show that coddled plants that never experience stressors like wind or brief droughts are actually weaker than plants that experience occasional discomfort. Good stressors like running a marathon, hiking a mountain, or giving a business presentation can actually make us feel better—depending on our perception.

What Happens During Stress

During moments of stress, a cascade of hormones is released.

These hormones course throughout the body and touch all organs and parts of the body. Our heart rates accelerate and blood pressure rises. Glucose is released to be used for quick energy. Hormones flood the body, some shutting down processes like digestion and suppressing sexual desire, while others increase strength, stamina, and speed.

Chronic Stress and Its Aftermath

The body is set up to handle stress the way nature defines stress. Think again about that saber tooth tiger. How often did our ancestors stumble upon a tiger in the forest? Once in a while perhaps, but most days our ancestors probably spent hunting, gathering, building homes, making tools, creating clothing, and caring for the basic necessities of life.

So then why does stress become a problem? First off, with our modern-day living, we face more chronic, long-term stress than our ancestors faced. Remember that the body is physiologically stressed when it is dehydrated. Often times people are in a state of chronic dehydration and therefore chronic stress. Chronic, long-term stress is destructive for many reasons:

- It keeps the body permanently on alert, with stress hormones, like cortisol, constantly high;
- There is rarely a moment when stress levels return to normal, let alone resting state; and
- Physiological markers become out of sync with the body's natural balance

Remember from earlier chapters that the human body always seeks to return to something called homeostasis, or balance. By constantly bombarding yourself with stress—either real or imaginary through things like worry—you put your body on a constant state of alertness that it was never intended to handle. You give no rest to the weary, so to speak. Think about your car. If you ran your car every day without changing the oil, the filters, inflating the tires and refueling it, what would happen? Pretty soon it would be a burned out shell sitting by the side of the road, not able to get you anywhere.

Scary picture, isn't it?

The Acidic Effects of Stress

Physically, chronic stress adds an additional acidic burden on the body. Chronic stress creates something called catabolism. Catabolism is a set of molecular pathways that break big molecules down into smaller ones. As the molecules break down, they release energy as well as byproducts such as lactic acid, acetic acid, carbon dioxide and urea. These wastes begin to build up and form what Dr. Peter Kopko, D.C. refers to as "slow death."

Shallow breathing—often a symptom of someone under stress—causes carbon dioxide accumulation in the blood. This causes a rise in acidity. Most people under chronic stress either stop perspiring, which means they are not excreting the toxins, or they perspire too much, which leads to dehydration. The stomach excretes more acid, and pro-inflammatory cytokines are released, which depresses the immune system and provides a hotbed for chronic inflammation to develop.

Keep in mind that all of these waste products circulate throughout the body, so all systems and organs can be affected by them. These toxins create an acidic environment.

So if you're eating a wonderfully alkaline diet, sipping your alkaline water, and you think you've got all bases covered…congratulations on taking charge of your health. But if you're immersed in daily stress or do not have healthy coping mechanisms in place, you'll end up with an additional acidic load to handle.

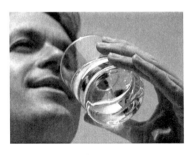

Stress Busters

So what can you do to mitigate all that stress?

There are myriad books, papers, CD ROMs, websites, gurus, teachers and courses to help you reduce stress. From tackling things on a very concrete level, like leaving home a few minutes earlier to avoid feeling stressed, to taking time to meditate and clear your mind of the day's turmoil, there are many ways to reduce stress.

Some of the healthy ways you can reduce stress and its accompanying toxic load without special books, teachers or equipment are:

- Practice deep breathing: Stress tends to make people take shallow breaths. Try consciously breathing in and out. Try breathing in, holding your breath for a count of 5 or 10, then slowly releasing the breath to a count of 5 or 10. The count should be comfortable for you—there's no set number. It merely helps you regulate your breathing. The next time you're stuck in traffic, try deep breathing.

- Exercise: Study after study shows that physical exercise, from simple walking to participation in team sports, helps reduce chronic stress. So make time for a simple 10 minute walk around the block or pop in an exercise tape. Your entire body will thank you.

  o Mindful exercise: Some exercises are especially good for stress reduction. Yoga, with its slow, gentle stretches and postures, breathing exercises, and emphasis on concentration, is great for stress relief. Another wonderful exercise for stress relief includes t'ai chi chuan or simply t'ai chi, which is often described as a combination of Yoga and meditation. Its flowing movements and slow, concentrated exercise combined with deep yet gentle breathing is an excellent stress relieving exercise. For both exercises, research has demonstrated a reduction in LDD ("bad" cholesterol) levels of as much as 20-26 milligrams in various studies.[27]

- Group support: Having a strong network of family, friends and community contacts is important for good mental health. Schedule a girl's night out or a guy's day with your friends. No matter how busy you are, making time for social support and fun activities is a great way to reduce stress.

- Nature: Nature has a soothing effect. Even if you live in the concrete jungle, simply including green plants in your office or apartment, stepping outside to a nearby park, or indulging in a trip to the suburbs to see a bit of green helps. From watching the sunrise to enjoying a thunderstorm, nature has a calming effect on stress.
- Enjoy the arts: Do you love to paint or draw? Sing or dance? Play an instrument? Participation in your favorite art, whether joining the community theater group or reading a good book, enlivens the spirit and quiets the mind. It's a great way to reduce stress
- Play with pets: Karen Allen, PhD., a researcher at the University of Buffalo, New York, conducted a study[28] with stock brokers who had high blood pressure. Among the stockbrokers, those who owned pets demonstrated lower blood pressure during stressful situations than those who did not own pets. At the conclusion of the study, many went out and got pets! Whether you own a dog, cat, snake, bird or fish, pets add joy and companionship. If you cannot own a pet, consider spending time with a friend's pets, visiting or volunteering at a shelter, or finding other ways to be around our furry friends.

- Meditation: Meditation quiets the mind. It can be religious in nature, although there are many forms that are secular and do not invoke God or gods. Meditation can be as simple as sitting quietly in a chair and allowing the mind to focus on the beats of the heart, or repeating a word or phrase such as peace, love, calm or the name of a deity. Many other meditation techniques are available if these do not work for you. Meditation has demonstrated the ability to lower heart rate and blood pressure, and acts as a great stress reliever.

- Prayer: Prayer and participation in a religion have been found to reduce stress for many. The group support and unconditional love people feel from their houses of worship helps mitigate some of the stressors of life.

If you're interested in learning more about these and other stress relief techniques, one great place to find many stress-busting ideas it the famous Mayo Clinic[26] Visit http://www.mayoclinic.com/health/exercise-and-stress/sr00036 for useful tips on reducing stress, adding meditation and physical exercise to your life, and leading a healthier life.

Conclusion

So many things in life are beyond our control. Yet what we put into our bodies and feed our minds and hearts is mostly within our control. We can choose our diet. We can order our days to include healthy activities like exercise, meditation, time with friends, and more. We can choose to live a healthy lifestyle.

So, choose to live your best today. You couldn't choose your parents and the genes you were born with. Perhaps up until today you didn't choose the healthiest lifestyle. But today is a new day. Just for today, just for the next 24 hours, put down the cigarettes, the donut and the coffee or that soft drink. Lace up your sneakers, get your water bottle, and take a walk in the fresh morning dew. Lift your face to the sky and breathe deep. Choose life; Choose health.

Be well.

Appendix: Resources

The following resources may be helpful in your researching into the acid-alkaline diet, raw and Vegan foods, and alkaline water.

Acid-Alkaline Diet

A good book on this topic is Young, Robert O. and Shelley. *The pH Miracle Diet.* AOL Time Warner Books.

Websites:
• Brigham and Womens Hospital provides an unbiased and fairly balanced viewpoint on the alkaline diet. Although skeptical, they acknowledge that in test tube studies, an alkaline diet does appear to reduce cancer growth: http://www.brighamandwomens.org/healtheweightforwomen/special_topics/intelihealth0506.aspx?subID=submenu1[27]

Raw and Vegan Foods

The raw and Vegan community online is the best place to get started.

• Raw People is comprehensive website on raw foods and holistic living: **www.RawPeople.com.**
• Karen Knowler is a raw food coach who offers many free, downloadable resources to get you started on your raw food journey: www.therawfoodcoach.com
• Angela Stokes was featured on CNN news after losing 162 pounds on a raw food diet. She shares her expertise here: **www.rawreform.com.**
• Dr. Ritamarie Loscalzo, raw food expert, nutritionist, health coach and women's fatigue expert: **www.drritamarie.com**.

Recommended books include:

• Boutenko, Victoria. *Green for Life*. Details Victoria's studies on green smoothies, and how these alkaline-rich beverages helped her study participants beat various illnesses.
• Rose, Natalie. *The Raw Food Detox Diet*. A simple way to get started eating raw, Vegan foods and gently ease your body through the transition.

Alkaline Water

- **www.LifeIonizers.com** Provides information on alkaline water and alkaline water machines.
- **http://ionza.co.nz/water-ionizer-wikipedia** Provides basic information on alkaline water.

Citations

1. Cancer Facts and Figures, 2008: American Cancer Society publication, accessed at **http://www.cancer.org/downloads/STT/2008CAFFfinalsecured.pdf**
2. ibid
3. Taken from **http://blog.healia.com/00300/top-10-most-common-types-cancer-diagnosed-us-women**
4. pH readings and references taken from **http://staff.jccc.net/PDECELL/chemistry/phscale.html**
5. American Journal of Epidemiology: **http://aje.oxfordjournals.org/cgi/content/abtract/133/8/801**. Although the study only reports the data, speculation is that diet is the contributing factor to the difference in osteoporosis rates.
6. **http://quotationsbook.com/quote/15316/**
7. Science Daily, March 4 2008: New Genetic Marker for Breast Cancer Found. **http://www.sciencedaily.com/releases/2008/03/080303190610.htm**
8. Web MD: **http://www.webmd.com/breast-cancer/news/20070320/high-fat-diet-linked-breast-cancer**
9. American Cancer Society, "Eat Right to Prevent Colorectal Cancer", **http://www.cancer.org/docroot/NWS/content/NWS_1_1x_Eat_Right_to_Prevent_Colorectal_Cancer.asp**
10. Young, Robert O and Young, Shelley Redford. The pH Miracle for Weight Loss: Balance Your Body Chemistry and Achieve Your Ideal Weight, Chapter 2
11. From the website Phytochemicals: **http://www.phytochemicals.info/**
12. Lypocene: **http://en.wikipedia.org/wiki/Lycopene**
13. Ann Wigmore Institute, Wheatgrass, accessed on May 22, 2009. **http://www.annwigmore.org/living_foods.html#wheatgrass**
14. Cancer Tutor, accessed on May 22, 2009. **http://www.cancertutor.com/Cancer/Wheatgrass.html**

15. Meyerowitz, Steve. Health Benefits of Sprouts. Accessed on May 22, 2009. Sprout Net, http://www.sproutnet.com/nutrition_of_sprouts.htm

16. Enzymes: **http://users.rcn.com/jkimball.ma.ultranet/BiologyPages/E/Enzymes.html**

17. Minich, Deanna M. and Bland, Jeffrey S, "Acid-Alkaline Balance: Role in Chronic Disease and Detoxification." Alternative Therapies, July/August 2007, Vol. 13. No 4. page 62

18. Myers, Dennis M.D., as quoted in Acid-Alkaline Balance in Your Body, **www.cancer-healing.com**

19. As quoted on **http://www.kangenwaterreport.com/139/**

20. The Diet Channel: **http://www.thedietchannel.com/Cancer-Prevention-Top-10-Cancer-Fighting-Foods.htm**

21. Both references are quoted by Dr. Andrew Weil at **http://www.drweil.com/drw/u/id/ART02708**

22. Dietician.com: **http://www.dietitian.com/protein.html**

23. Ask a Healer: **http://www.askahealer.com/reverse-osmosis.htm**

24. Young, Dr. Robert O., *The pH Miracle for Weight Loss*. New York: Grand Central Publishing, 2005, pp. 65-68

25. Cancer Tutor, **http://www.cancertutor.com/Cancer/IonizedWater.html**

26. Brody, Jane. "Cutting Cholesterol: An Uphill Battle." The New York Times, August 21, 2007. Accessed at: **http://www.nytimes.com/2007/08/21/ health/21brod. html?_r=1&adxnnl=1&adxnnlx=1190862080-FWYKVQhkU70Kz/P+y3V9pw**

27. Medicine Net, **http://www.medicinenet.com/script/main/art.asp?articlekey=52360**

28. Mayo Clinic **http://www.mayoclinic.com/health/exercise-and-stress/sr00036**